Healing Teas for Wellness

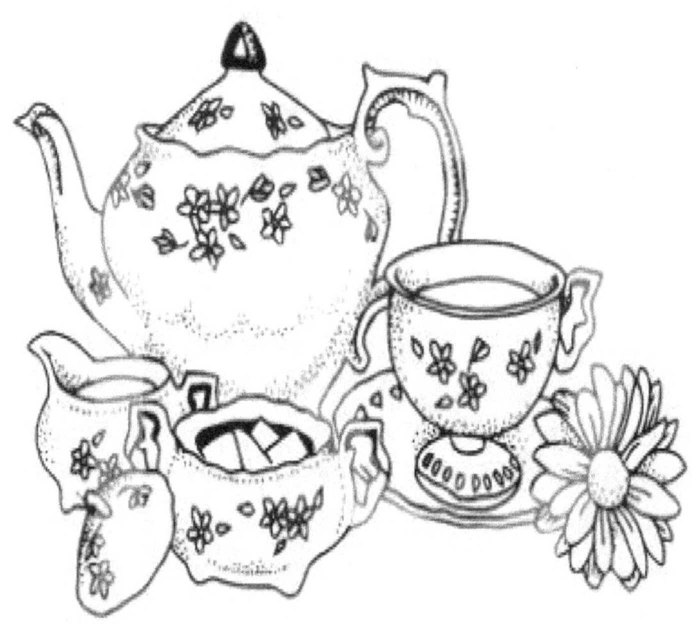

By: Janet Balletta

Healing Teas for Wellness

© 2020 by Janet Balletta

ISBN-13: 978-1679700651

Healing Teas for Wellness

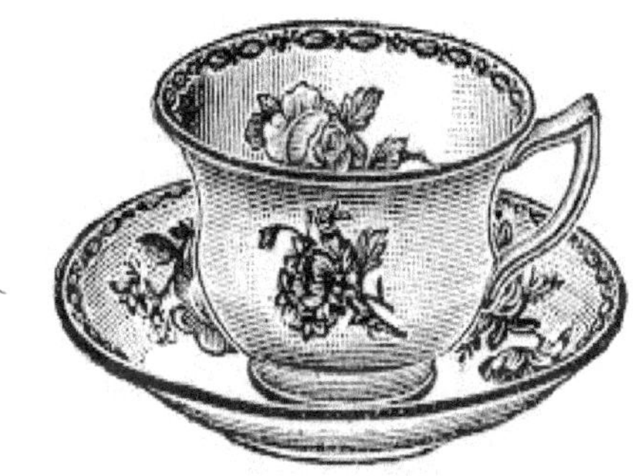

Dedication

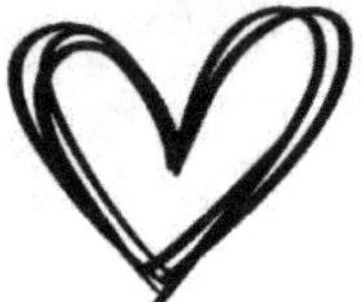

For my beloved family who support me in

my natural and holistic approach to healing the

body for living a healthy life.

Table of Contents

History of Tea

The history of tea is long and complex, spreading across multiple cultures over the span of thousands of years. Tea or *Camellia Sinensis* originated as a medicinal drink in the Yunnan region of China.

One popular Chinese Legend, Shennong, the legendary Emperor of China and inventor of agriculture and Chinese medicine was drinking a bowl of just boiled water due to a decree that his subjects must boil water before drinking it.

Around 2737 BC, a few leaves were blown, from a nearby tree, into his water, changing the color and taste. The emperor took a sip of the brew and was pleasantly surprised by its flavor and restorative properties.

Another version of the legend claims the emperor tested the medical properties of various herbs on himself, some of them poisonous, and found tea to work as an antidote. Shennong is also mentioned in Lu Yu's famous early work on the subject, *The Classic of Tea*.

A similar Chinese legend goes that the god of agriculture would chew the leaves, stems, and roots of various plants to discover medicinal herbs. If he consumed a poisonous plant, he would chew tea leaves to counteract the poison.

Today, tea, is popular around the world and used for its medicinal properties, health benefits, and calming effects. As a lifelong tea lover, I enjoy sharing teas that help with a variety of ailments. Moreover, tea soothes your body, mind, and soul so your body can heal naturally.

Anise Star Tea

Anise star tea is the seed pod from the fruit of the Illicium verum plant native to China. It's famous for its medicinal properties. Anise star tea is rich in antioxidants and vitamin A and C which help fight free radicals that are responsible for early aging and diabetes. The oil produced from Anise contains thymol, terpineol and anethole, which is used for treating cough and flu. Anise star tea also helps improve digestion, alleviate cramps, and reduce nausea. Drinking Anise tea after meals helps treat digestive ailments such as bloating, gas, indigestion, and constipation.

Black Tea

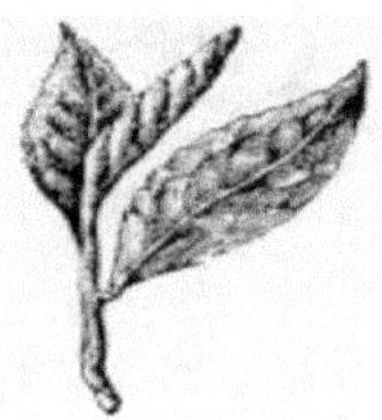

Black tea is cultivated in Asia. It's stronger than regular teas because it's more oxidized and has numerous health benefits. It's loaded with antioxidants called polyphenols that protect human cells from hazardous free radical damage. Black tea makes the top anti-aging foods list as it has been linked with improved mental alertness, lower ovarian cancer risk, and a decreased chance of developing Parkinson's disease, diabetes, and heart disease. Black tea has a lot of caffeine so don't drink more than two cups a day as it may cause insomnia and anxiety.

Chamomile Tea

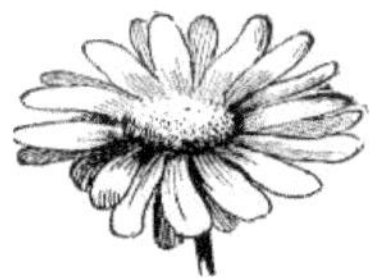

Chamomile tea originated in Egypt. It's an herb that comes from the daisy flowers of the Asteraceae plant family. Chamomile tea has been used for hundreds of years for lots of health conditions. It's known for its sweet taste and is a great caffeine-free alternative to black or green tea. Chamomile tea is loaded with antioxidants which helps lower risk of heart disease and cancer. Chamomile tea is used for digestion, sleep, and menstrual cramps.

Chai Tea

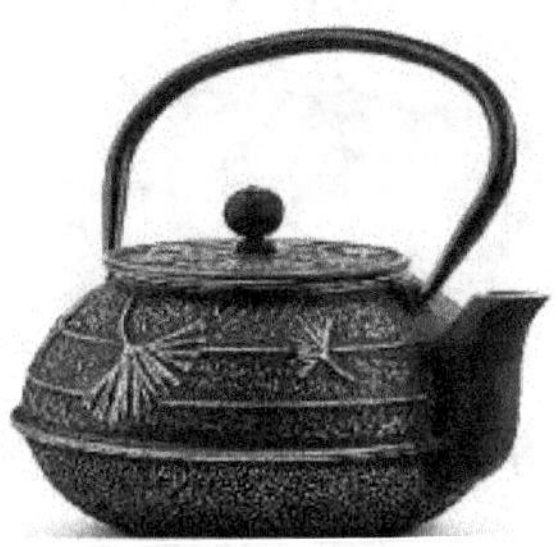

Chai (Masala) tea originated in India. Chai tea is made by brewing black tea, milk, and a mixture of cardamon, fresh ginger, black pepper, ground cloves, cinnamon and fennel. Chai tea has more polyphenols than fruits and vegetables. It has become a worldwide tea featured in many tea houses. Chai tea is good for sleep, lowers blood pressure, digestion, reduces risk of cancer, and maintains a healthy heart.

Cistus Incanus Tea

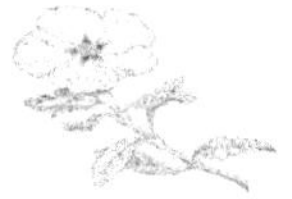

Cistus Incanus tea is native to the Mediterranean. It comes from a flower with purple and pink petals and considered the new miracle tea. It's known for treating strep throat, upper respiratory infections, cancer, HIV, and many other retroviruses. The tea is popular in Italy but gaining popularity in the United States for its amazing curative properties. The principal active constituents of the Cistus are polyphenols which have been shown to be strong antioxidants with numerous health benefits including anti-aging, detoxing from Candida, biofilms, and whitens teeth naturally.

Dandelion Tea

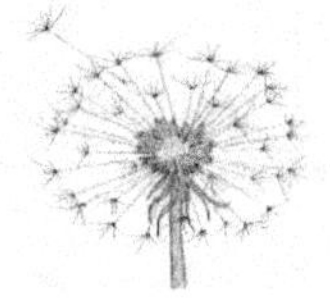

Dandelion tea is native to Greece. It contains Vitamin A, natural anti-inflammatory, and antioxidant properties. In Greece, people eat dandelion greens in salads called Horta. Dandelion tea helps the kidneys, liver, and gallbladder. It's a natural diuretic which means it encourages urination, prevents urinary tract infections, and water retention. Studies show it lowers cholesterol in animals but is still being researched for its effects on humans. Dandelion tea also fights the flu and shortens the duration of the flu. So, drink or eat Dandelions to improve your health.

Elm (Slippery) Tea

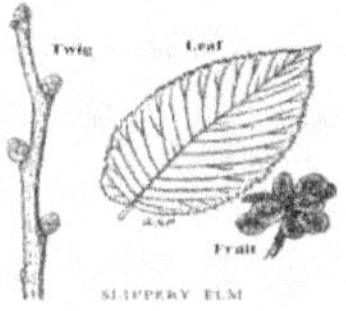

Elm (Slippery) tea comes from the inner bark of trees grown in the Adirondacks and many parts of the U.S. Elm tea is used for its medicinal purposes in syrup or tea for coughs, sore throats, colic, diarrhea, constipation, hemorrhoids, irritable bowel syndrome, (IBS), bladder, urinary tract infections, syphilis, herpes, and for expelling tapeworms. It is also used for protecting against stomach and duodenal ulcers, for colitis, diverticulitis, GI inflammation, heartburn, and acid reflux.

Fennel Tea

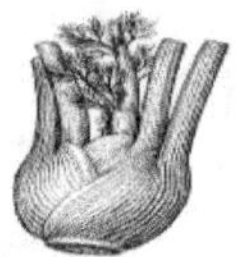

Fennel tea is native to Asia and Europe but is also grown in many parts of the United States. It comes from the seeds of a crunchy, pale-green root and carrot top-like fronds. Fennel tea was first used by the Roman naturalist Pliny who lived from 23 to 79 AD. King Edward also used fennel tea as a condiment and appetite suppressant for the purpose of fasting. Fennel tea was brought to the United States by the Puritans. It promotes healthy digestion, is a diuretic, helps relax muscles of the gastrointestinal system, reduces gas, bloating, and stomach cramps. Many people like its natural, sweet licorice taste.

Ginger Tea

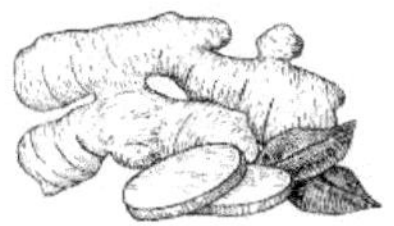

Ginger tea comes from a plant of the Zingiberaceae family in Asia. Ginger tea is made from the root or stem and used as a herbal remedy for many ailments. Drinking ginger tea cures everything from motion sickness to cancer prevention. Experts believe the volatile oils and phenol compounds called gingerols help relieve nausea caused by pregnancy, chemotherapy, or surgery. (Check with a doctor before using ginger after surgery, as it may interfere with clotting.) Ginger also lowers blood pressure, cholesterol, prevents heart attack, and increases blood circulation. It's used to induce labor as well.

Hibiscus Tea

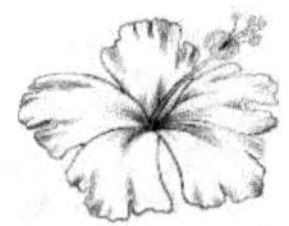

Hibiscus tea originated in Asia where it has been used for centuries for its medicinal purposes. It can be served cold or hot. Hibiscus tea has been known to prevent hypertension, lower blood pressure, reduce blood sugar levels, keep your liver healthy, help with menstrual cramps, help with depression, aid digestion, and help with weight management. It's rich in Vitamin C, contains minerals such as flavonoids, and has natural laxative properties. Hibiscus tea has become so popular on the Keto diet for weight loss that Starbucks added the Pink Tea.

Kombucha Tea

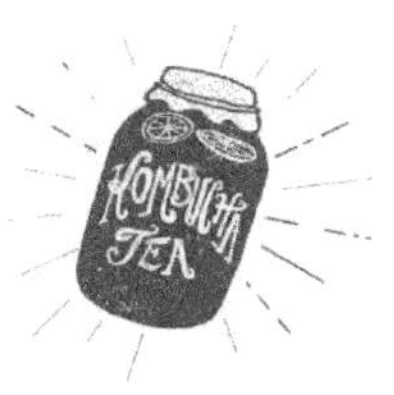

Kombucha tea originated in Japan and has been around for roughly 2000 years. Kombucha tea is made from brown seaweed or kelp. It's a lightly sweetened, fermented tea (usually black tea or sometimes **green tea** is used). It contains a colony of bacteria and yeast which is responsible for the fermented process once combined with sugar. The benefits of Kombucha tea is increased **healthy bacteria in the digestive system and immune function.** The probiotics in Kombucha improve gut health and strengthen the immune system.

Lemongrass Tea

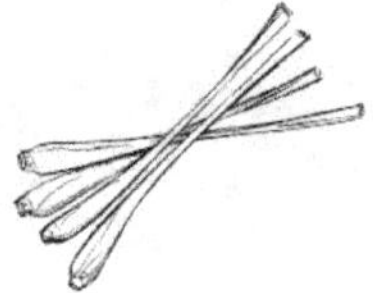

Lemongrass tea comes from an herb native to Sri Lanka and South India, but now grows in many countries around the world. The plant's stalks are a common ingredient in Asian cooking, but it is also used to brew Lemongrass tea. The benefits of Lemongrass tea are numerous. This tea is known to alleviate stress and anxiety, lower cholesterol, prevent infection, relieve pain and bloating, boost oral health, and red blood cell formation.

Matcha Tea

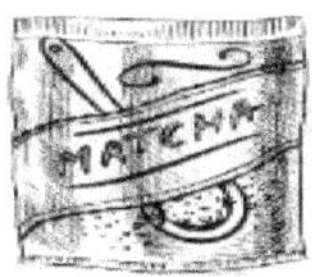

Matcha Green tea originated in Japan, and because the entire leaf is ingested in powder form, it is the most potent green tea in the world. In Japanese "cha" means tea, and "ma" means powder, so the word matcha translates as powdered green tea. Matcha tea contains a unique, potent class of antioxidant known as catechins, which aren't found in other foods. The catechin EGCg (epigallocatechin gallate) provides potent cancer-fighting properties. EGCg and other catechins counteract the effects free radicals from pollution, UV rays, radiation, and chemicals, which can lead to cell and DNA damage.

Moringa Tea

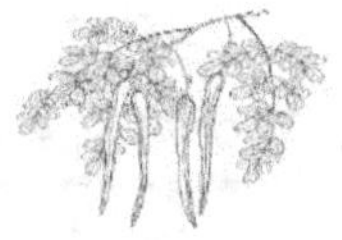

Moringa tea comes from a tree native to India but also grows in Asia, Africa, and South America. Moringa tea has been used for centuries for its health benefits. It contains a variety of proteins, vitamins, and minerals such as vitamin A, vitamin B1, B2, B3, B-6, folate acid and ascorbic acid, vitamin C, calcium, potassium, iron, magnesium, phosphorus, and zinc. It's packed with antioxidants needed for a healthy heart. It has antifungal, antiviral, and anti-inflammatory properties. Moringa tea helps lower blood pressure and reduces asthma attacks as it protects the bronchioles and lungs.

Nettle Tea

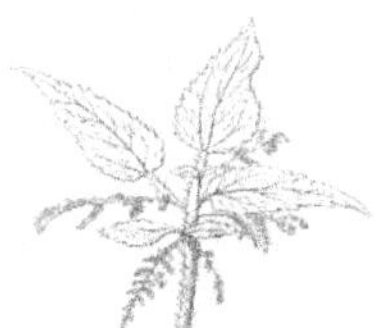

Nettle tea comes from the Stinging Nettle flower which grows wild in temperate regions around the world. Nettle tea is packed with vitamins, minerals, and potent phytonutrients including deep-green chlorophyll. The leaves have more minerals, especially magnesium and calcium, than many other medicinal herbs. Nettle tea is a gentle diuretic, helping the body to process and flush away toxins. It flushes the kidneys and bladder to prevent and soothe urinary tract infections. Nettle tea is also known to support healthy joints according to the Arthritis Foundation.

Oolong Tea

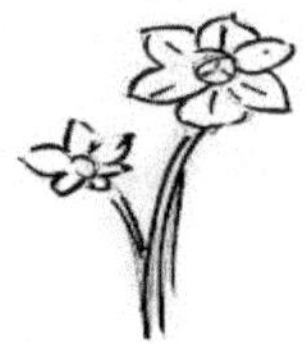

Oolong tea comes from China. The word Oolong is made up of two words "black" and "dragon." Its name describes the shape of the leaves. Oolong teas vary in flavor. They can be sweet and fruity with honey aromas, or woody and thick with roasted aromas, or green and fresh with complex aromas. Oolong tea has a variety of benefits including heart, brain, bone and dental health. In addition, it may boost your metabolism, decrease your risk of developing type 2 diabetes and protect against certain types of cancer. Oolong tea has lots of Caffeine too so don't drink it too much or it may produce insomnia and anxiety.

Parsley Tea

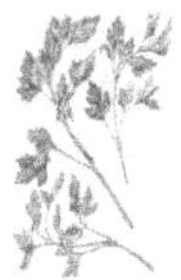

Parsley tea is native to the Mediterranean region. It's packed with flavonoids and antioxidants like luteolin, lycopene, folic acid, Vitamin A, Vitamin C, and Vitamin K. Parsley tea has many health benefits including controlling blood sugar levels, preventing kidney stones, regulating menstruation, blocking cancer cells, and protecting against infections like pneumonia. It's also involved in the synthesis of collagen the protein required for healthy skin, bones, tendons, and joints. Pregnant women should not drink parsley tea as it can induce miscarriages.

Quinine (Wild) Tea

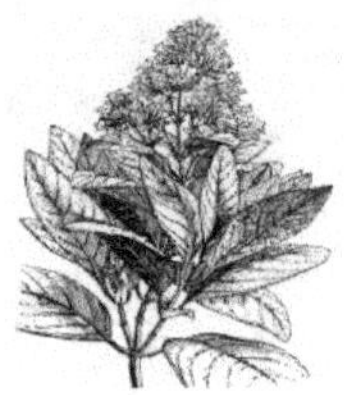

Quinine (Wild) tea or cinchona is one of the rainforest's most famous plants and most important discoveries. The name cinchona came from the countess of Chinchon, the wife of a Peruvian viceroy, who was cured of malaria fever by using the bark of the cinchona tree. Quinine tea is making a big come back for its curative power against malaria, restless legs syndrome, and leg cramps. Quinine tea can be used to fight many infections like bronchitis, colitis, Crohn's disease, as well as chronic inflammatory diseases.

Sage Tea

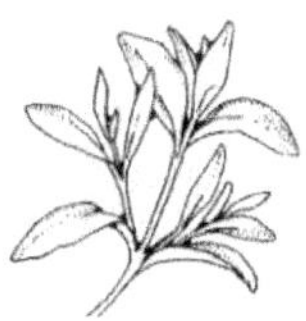

Sage tea has a rich history due to both its medicinal and culinary uses. At one time, the French produced bountiful crops of sage which they used as a tea. The Chinese became enamored with French sage tea, trading four pounds of Chinese tea for every one pound of sage tea. Sage tea is loaded with antioxidants that are linked to better health. Chlorogenic acid, caffeic acid, rosmarinus acid, ellagic acid, and Rutin all found in sage are linked to impressive benefits, such as a lower risk of cancer, improved brain function, and memory. In addition, sage tea, is used to relieve menopause symptoms.

Turmeric Tea

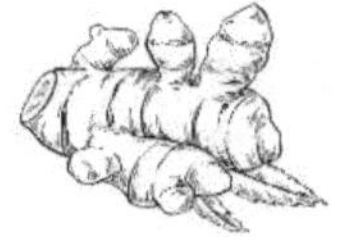

Turmeric tea comes from a perennial rhizomatous herb belonging to the Zingiberaceae family which originated in India. It also has a long history of medicinal uses in Asia. Now Turmeric is widely cultivated in tropical as well as subtropical regions around the globe. More commonly known as the golden spice used in curry and now recognized worldwide as a superfood. Turmeric tea has strong anti-inflammatory properties can help ease inflammation and pain in people with arthritis, osteoarthritis, and respiratory diseases like pneumonia and asthma.

White Tea

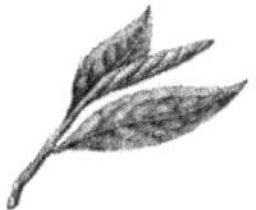

White tea originated in China during the Chinese Imperial Dynasties (600-1300). During the Song Dynasty (960-1297), the young tea buds would be plucked, meticulously rinsed, and ground into a white powder. White tea is packed with antioxidants, which makes it an incredibly healthy tea. Compared to Green tea, white tea is less processed, retains higher amounts of antioxidants, and has less caffeine, therefore, white tea is a healthier choice. Studies have linked white tea to impressive health benefits, including a lower risk of heart disease, and cancer. It may also help with weight loss.

Yerba Mate

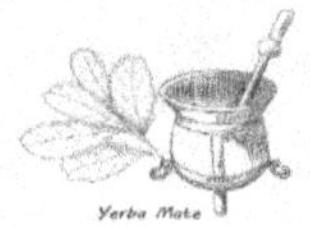

Yerba Mate tea is made from the leaves of the Ilex Paraguariensis plant. The plant is grown and processed in South   America, Argentina,   Paraguay, Uruguay and Brazil. Yerba   Mate   tea   contains   caffeine, theobromine, antioxidants, and polyphenols. It lowers cholesterol, and blood sugars to regulate diabetes, reduces risk of cancer, and boosts the immune system and metabolism for weight management. Yerba mate tea is traditionally served in a container called a gourd, also known as a calabash. It's commonly sipped through a metal straw that has a filter on the bottom to strain out the leaf fragments.

My Tea Healing Journey

My tea healing journey evolved over the years. I was not allowed to drink coffee as child, although it's a common practice among Hispanics. When I was young, my mother gave me **Anise tea** for an upset stomach and **Chamomile tea** for menstrual cramps. At the age of thirteen, I became a tea lover after a friend introduced me to drinking tea daily.

As an adult, I suffered with asthma, digestion issues, and acid reflux. **Slippery Elm and Fennel tea** became my go-to teas to treat digestion problems and reduce acid reflux. Years ago, I had a terrible bout of pneumonia and tried **Turmeric tea**. After one week, I was cured! I continued using Turmeric tea for its anti-inflammatory benefits to control my asthma.

Recently, I had pelvic surgery and used **Cistus Incanus tea** to aid my recovery and cleanse my body of anesthesia, antibiotics, and medications. I recommend Cistus Incanus tea for anyone having surgery. Not only does it accelerate your healing time, but it detoxes your body in the process.

Sage is my preferred tea to keep the menopause symptoms at bay. It works wonders for insomnia, hot flashes, and weight management. I also use **Green tea** and **Hibiscus tea** for weight loss. They suppress my appetite for hours.

When I feel a cold coming on, I drink a cup of **Dandelion tea** with cinnamon and honey. It strengthens my immune system to fight the cold, virus, or flu.

In fact, even if I get sick the duration of the cold is shortened.

Finally, inform your doctors of any teas you use as natural remedies to make sure they don't interact with any of your medications.

You can transform your life by getting healthy and fit with *Healing Teas for Wellness*. Here's to a healthier new you in 2020!

Tea Haiku

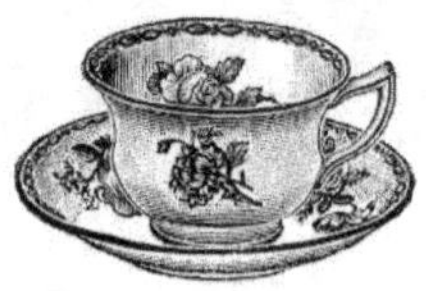

Morning by morning

Sipping tea in gratitude

Honoring our God

Children's Books

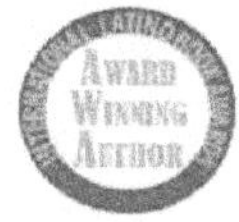
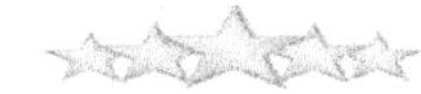
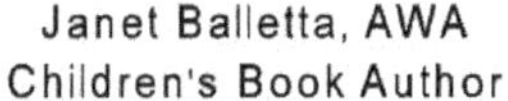
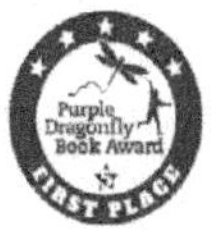

Janet Balletta, AWA
Children's Book Author

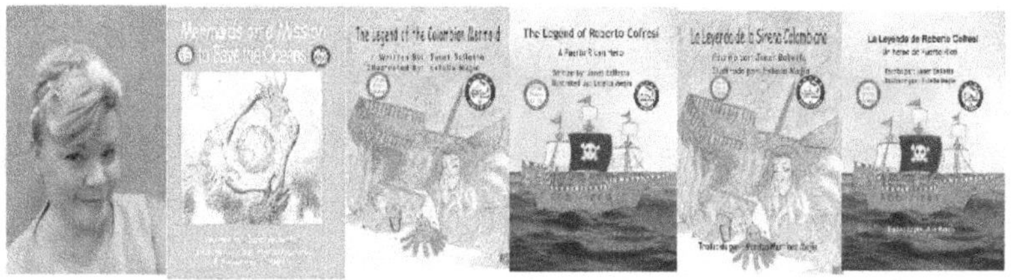

The Legend of the Colombian Mermaid is a magical story with themes of
obedience, family values, and cultural traditions. For Ages 5-12

The Legend of Roberto Cofresi - A Puerto Rican Hero is an enchanting story with themes of
generosity, loyalty, and cultural traditions. For Ages 5-12

Mermaids on a Mission to Save the Oceans is an innovative story with themes of
environmental awareness, water pollution, and conservation. For Ages 5 -12

www.amazon.com/Janet-Balletta/e/B00HZ9QEYK
Visit my website janetballetta.com for free learning activities.

www.ingramcontent.com/pod-product-compliance
Lightning Source LLC
Chambersburg PA
CBHW050710250726
48662CB00002B/940